ADDUCTOR MASSAGE

TECHNIQUES

A Comprehensive Guide To Relieving Inner Thigh Pain, Improving Mobility, And Enhancing Athletic Performance Through Deep Tissue Massage And Myofascial Release

ROBERT LUGO

CHAPTER 1
Introduction To Adductor Muscles

The adductor muscles are a group of muscles located in the inner thigh region of the body. Understanding their anatomy, functions, and common issues is crucial for effective adductor massage techniques.

Anatomy of the Adductor Muscles: The adductor muscles consist of several individual muscles that work together to perform adduction, which is the movement of bringing the legs toward the midline of the body. These muscles include the adductor longus, adductor brevis, adductor magnus, gracilis, and pectineus. They originate from different points on the pelvis and femur and are inserted along the femur and the pelvis.

The adductor magnus, for instance, has two parts: the adductor part and the hamstring part, each with distinct functions.

Understanding the specific attachments and actions of each muscle helps in targeting them effectively during massage.

Functions and Importance in Movement: The adductor muscles play a crucial role in various movements of the lower body.

Their primary function is adduction, which is essential for activities like walking, running, and jumping. Additionally, these muscles contribute to stability and balance during movements involving lateral shifts or changes in direction.

They work in coordination with other muscles of the hip and thigh to maintain proper alignment and joint function. Weakness or tightness in the adductors can lead to imbalances, affecting overall movement efficiency and increasing the risk of injuries.

Common Issues and Injuries Associated with Adductors: One common issue related to the adductor muscles is tightness or stiffness, often caused by prolonged sitting, lack of stretching, or improper exercise techniques.

Tight adductors can restrict the range of motion and lead to discomfort or pain, especially during activities that require wide leg movements.

On the other hand, weakness in the adductors can result from underuse or inadequate strength training, leading to instability and increased susceptibility to strains or tears, particularly during sudden movements or high-impact activities.

Injuries to the adductor muscles are prevalent among athletes, especially those involved in sports that require quick changes in direction or explosive movements. Adductor strains, characterized by pain and tenderness in the inner thigh, are common in sports like soccer, basketball, and hockey. Overuse injuries, such as tendinitis or bursitis, can also occur due to repetitive motions or excessive stress on the adductors without adequate rest or recovery.

Understanding the anatomy, functions, and potential issues associated with the adductor muscles is fundamental for developing effective massage techniques aimed at relieving tension, improving flexibility, and promoting overall lower body health and performance.

CHAPTER 2
Benefits Of Adductor Massage

Adductor massage techniques offer a range of benefits that contribute significantly to overall physical well-being and athletic performance.

One of the key advantages of adductor massage is the improvement in flexibility and range of motion. This is especially beneficial for individuals engaged in activities that require a wide range of leg movements, such as dancers, athletes, and fitness enthusiasts.

By targeting the adductor muscles, which are responsible for bringing the legs toward the midline of the body, massage helps to loosen tight muscles and improve their elasticity. This increased flexibility not only enhances performance but also reduces the risk of injuries related to limited range of motion.

Moreover, adductor massage plays a crucial role in reducing muscle tension and pain.

The adductor muscles can become tight and knotted due to various factors such as overuse, poor posture, or inadequate warm-up before physical activity.

This tightness can lead to discomfort, stiffness, and even pain in the groin area and inner thighs. Through targeted massage techniques, such as deep tissue massage or myofascial release, tension and knots in the adductor muscles can be alleviated. This not only provides immediate relief from pain but also promotes better muscle function and overall comfort.

Another significant benefit of adductor massage is its impact on enhancing athletic performance and preventing injuries. Athletes, in particular, can benefit greatly from regular adductor massage as it helps to improve muscle efficiency and coordination. When the adductor muscles are free from tension and knots, they can contract and relax more effectively, allowing for smoother and more powerful movements during physical activities.

This, in turn, can lead to enhanced performance in sports that require agility, speed, and explosive movements.

Furthermore, adductor massage contributes to injury prevention by addressing underlying muscle imbalances and weaknesses. Imbalances in the adductor muscles, where certain muscles are stronger or more active than others, can lead to biomechanical issues and increase the risk of injuries such as strains or pulls.

Through targeted massage techniques and corrective exercises, these imbalances can be addressed, leading to better muscle symmetry and reduced injury risk.

the benefits of adductor massage are multifaceted and impactful. From improving flexibility and range of motion to reducing muscle tension and enhancing athletic performance, adductor massage techniques offer a holistic approach to optimizing physical well-being and supporting long-term fitness goals. Incorporating regular adductor massage into a comprehensive training and recovery regimen can yield significant benefits for individuals across various fitness levels and athletic pursuits.

CHAPTER 3
Understanding Massage Techniques

Understanding massage techniques involves delving into the basics of massage therapy, understanding specific considerations for adductor massage, and exploring different types of massage strokes and their effects. Massage therapy encompasses a range of manual techniques aimed at manipulating soft tissues to promote relaxation, reduce muscle tension, alleviate pain, improve circulation, and enhance overall well-being.

These techniques are rooted in anatomical knowledge and therapeutic principles, making them valuable tools in addressing various musculoskeletal issues.

Adductor massage, in particular, focuses on the adductor muscles located on the inner thigh. These muscles play a crucial role in hip stability, leg movement, and overall lower body function. Specific considerations come into play when performing adductor massage due to the sensitive nature of these muscles and their susceptibility to tightness, strain, and injury. Understanding the anatomy and function of the adductor muscles is essential for effective and safe massage therapy.

Different types of massage strokes are utilized in adductor massage, each with distinct effects on the tissues and therapeutic outcomes. Effleurage involves gentle, gliding strokes that help warm up the muscles and improve circulation. Petrissage utilizes kneading and squeezing motions to target deeper layers of muscle tissue and release tension. Friction involves firm pressure and circular movements to break down adhesions and improve mobility.

Tapotement includes rhythmic tapping or percussive strokes that stimulate the muscles and promote relaxation.

The choice of massage stroke depends on the client's needs, preferences, and the therapist's assessment of the adductor muscles' condition.

A combination of strokes may be used to achieve optimal results, such as relieving tightness, enhancing flexibility, reducing pain, and improving range of motion. Proper technique, pressure, and pacing are crucial aspects of adductor massage to ensure effectiveness and prevent potential discomfort or injury.

In addition to hands-on techniques, adductor massage may incorporate other modalities such as stretching, heat therapy, and corrective exercises. Stretching exercises targeting the adductor muscles can complement massage therapy by further releasing tension and improving flexibility. Heat therapy, through methods like hot packs or warm towels, can help relax the muscles and enhance the effects of massage. Corrective exercises focus on strengthening and stabilizing the adductor muscles to prevent future issues and support long-term musculoskeletal health.

Overall, understanding massage techniques for the adductor muscles involves a comprehensive approach that integrates anatomical knowledge, therapeutic principles, and tailored interventions. By combining different massage strokes, adjunct therapies, and client-centered care, therapists can effectively address adductor-related issues, improve muscular function, and promote overall well-being for their clients.

CHAPTER 4
Preparing For Adductor Massage

When preparing for adductor massage, it's crucial to start by assessing the individual's needs and goals. This assessment involves understanding the specific issues or discomfort the person is experiencing related to their adductor muscles. For some, it could be tightness or soreness from physical activities or a sedentary lifestyle.

Others may seek massage to improve flexibility or address chronic pain in the adductor region. By identifying these needs and goals, the massage therapist can tailor the session to focus on areas that require attention and deliver effective results.

Creating a comfortable environment is essential for a successful adductor massage session. This involves setting up a relaxing space that promotes a sense of calm and tranquility.

The massage room should be quiet, with soft lighting and soothing music to enhance relaxation. Comfortable massage tables or chairs with appropriate cushioning can help the client feel at ease during the session. Additionally, providing blankets or towels for warmth and privacy contributes to a comfortable environment conducive to effective massage therapy.

Safety precautions and contraindications play a vital role in adductor massage to ensure the client's well-being. Before starting the massage, the therapist should inquire about any medical conditions, injuries, or areas of sensitivity that could impact the session. This information helps the therapist avoid techniques or pressure that may cause discomfort or exacerbate existing issues. For example, clients with certain medical conditions like deep vein thrombosis or recent surgeries may have contraindications for massage on their adductors, requiring modifications or alternative approaches for treatment.

Understanding the client's medical history and current health status is crucial for implementing appropriate safety measures during adductor massage. The therapist should be aware of any allergies, skin sensitivities, or medications that could affect the massage session. Clear communication with the client about their comfort level, pain tolerance, and feedback during the massage helps ensure a safe and effective experience. Regularly checking in with the client and adjusting techniques as needed based on their response contributes to a positive and beneficial massage outcome.

CHAPTER 5
Techniques For Adductor Massage

Effleurage and petrissage strokes are fundamental techniques used in adductor massage to enhance flexibility, relieve tension, and improve overall muscle function. Effleurage involves long, sweeping strokes applied with moderate pressure using the palms of the hands. This technique is often used at the beginning of a massage session to warm up the muscles, increase blood flow, and prepare the adductors for deeper work. Petrissage, on the other hand, involves kneading, lifting, and squeezing motions that target specific areas of tension within the adductor muscles. By alternating between effleurage and petrissage strokes, massage therapists can effectively address tightness and promote relaxation in the adductors.

Myofascial release techniques play a crucial role in adductor massage by targeting the fascia, a connective tissue that surrounds and supports muscles, to release tension and improve mobility.

One common myofascial release technique is the use of sustained pressure on trigger points or areas of tightness within the adductors. This pressure helps to break up adhesions and knots in the fascia, allowing for greater flexibility and range of motion. Additionally, myofascial stretching techniques may be incorporated to further lengthen and loosen the adductor muscles, promoting optimal function and reducing the risk of injury.

Deep tissue massage is another effective approach for addressing adductor tightness and discomfort. This technique involves applying firm pressure and slow, deliberate strokes to target the deeper layers of muscle tissue. By focusing on the adductor group's deep muscles, such as the adductor longus, adductor brevis, and adductor magnus, deep tissue massage can help release chronic tension, improve circulation, and restore proper muscle function. Massage therapists need to communicate with clients during deep tissue work to ensure the pressure is comfortable and effective in addressing specific areas of concern within the adductors.

Incorporating effleurage and petrissage strokes, myofascial release techniques, and deep tissue massage into an adductor massage session can yield significant benefits in terms of flexibility, pain relief, and overall muscle health.

These techniques work synergistically to target different layers of muscle tissue and promote optimal function, making them valuable tools for addressing adductor tightness and improving athletic performance.

CHAPTER 6
Special Considerations

When delving into adductor massage techniques, it's crucial to consider the special aspects that can enhance the effectiveness and safety of these practices. One area of focus is the utilization of massage tools and equipment.

These tools can vary widely, from simple handheld devices like foam rollers and massage balls to more advanced equipment such as percussion massagers or vibrating foam rollers. The choice of tools depends on factors like the intensity of massage desired, the specific muscles targeted within the adductor group, and the individual's comfort level and physical condition.

Incorporating stretching and mobility exercises alongside adductor massage is another vital consideration. Massage alone can improve blood flow, release tension, and promote relaxation in the muscles. However, combining it with stretching and mobility exercises can further enhance flexibility, range of motion, and overall muscle function. Dynamic stretching, static stretching, and mobility drills tailored to the adductor muscles can be integrated into a comprehensive massage therapy session to address both soft tissue tightness and joint mobility.

Furthermore, the integration of massage with other therapeutic modalities can offer comprehensive benefits. Techniques such as heat therapy, cold therapy, or contrast therapy (alternating between hot and cold applications) can complement adductor massage by reducing inflammation, alleviating pain, and accelerating recovery. Additionally, incorporating modalities like electrotherapy (e.g., TENS units) or myofascial release techniques can further enhance the outcomes of adductor massage, especially in cases of chronic muscle tightness or injury rehabilitation.

By considering these special aspects—utilizing appropriate massage tools and equipment, integrating stretching and mobility exercises, and combining massage with other complementary therapies—adductor massage techniques can be optimized for maximum effectiveness and tailored to individual needs, whether for athletic performance enhancement, injury prevention, or general well-being.

CHAPTER 7
Post-Massage Care

Post-massage care is crucial for maximizing the benefits of adductor massage techniques. Hydration and nutrition play a significant role in supporting muscle recovery and overall well-being. Adequate hydration is essential to help flush out toxins released during the massage and maintain optimal muscle function.

It's recommended to drink plenty of water throughout the day, especially after a massage session, to replenish lost fluids and aid in the healing process.

In addition to hydration, nutrition plays a vital role in post-massage care. Consuming a balanced diet rich in nutrients such as protein, vitamins, and minerals supports muscle repair and growth. Including foods high in antioxidants can also help reduce inflammation and promote faster recovery.

Nutrient-dense foods like lean proteins, fruits, vegetables, whole grains, and healthy fats are beneficial for overall muscle health and recovery after adductor massage sessions.

Rest and recovery are equally important aspects of post-massage care. Giving the muscles adequate time to rest allows them to heal and adapt to the massage therapy.

It's essential to listen to your body's signals and avoid overexertion or intense physical activity immediately after a massage. Incorporating rest days into your workout routine helps prevent muscle fatigue and reduces the risk of injury, allowing for better recovery and long-term progress.

Monitoring progress and adjusting techniques are essential for optimizing the benefits of adductor massage. Keeping track of how your muscles respond to massage therapy helps determine the effectiveness of the techniques used.

If you notice improvements in flexibility, reduced muscle tension, or enhanced range of motion, it indicates that the massage techniques are beneficial.

On the other hand, if you experience persistent discomfort or limited progress, it may be necessary to adjust the massage techniques or seek guidance from a professional massage therapist.

Regularly assessing your massage sessions' outcomes and making necessary adjustments ensures that you continue to derive maximum benefits from adductor massage techniques.

Whether it's modifying pressure levels, exploring different massage strokes, or incorporating additional stretching exercises, adapting your approach based on progress monitoring enhances the overall effectiveness of the massage therapy.

Post-massage care plays a critical role in maximizing the benefits of adductor massage techniques.

Hydration and nutrition support muscle recovery, while rest and recovery strategies allow for optimal healing and adaptation. Monitoring progress and adjusting techniques based on outcomes ensure ongoing improvement and long-term success in incorporating adductor massage into your wellness routine.

CHAPTER 8
Advanced Techniques And Adaptations

Advanced techniques in adductor massage involve a nuanced understanding of the musculature involved, as well as adaptations tailored to specific needs such as sports, rehabilitation, and long-term maintenance.

In sports-specific adductor massage, the focus extends beyond general techniques to address the unique demands of athletes. This includes considering the types of movements and stresses typical in the athlete's sport, such as the rapid lateral movements in soccer or the explosive power required in weightlifting. Techniques may be modified to target not just the adductors but also surrounding muscles crucial for athletic performance and injury prevention.

Rehabilitation protocols for adductor injuries require a multifaceted approach.

Initially, the emphasis is on reducing inflammation and pain while promoting tissue healing. This may involve gentle massage techniques aimed at improving circulation and lymphatic drainage. As the healing process advances, more specialised methods like deep tissue massage and myofascial release massage can be incorporated to address scar tissue and restore flexibility and strength.

Long-term maintenance and preventive strategies in adductor massage are essential for athletes and individuals prone to adductor strains. This involves regular sessions focused on maintaining optimal muscle length and flexibility, addressing imbalances that can lead to injuries, and incorporating corrective exercises and stretches into the client's routine. Prevention also includes education on proper warm-up techniques, biomechanics, and training modifications to reduce the risk of adductor injuries over time.

CHAPTER 9
Case Studies And Success Stories

Case studies and success stories offer compelling evidence of the effectiveness of adductor massage techniques in addressing various issues related to the adductor muscles. By delving into real-life examples, we can uncover the tangible benefits experienced by clients, understand their journey, and extract valuable lessons and practical applications for adductor massage therapies.

In exploring real-life examples of adductor massage benefits, we encounter individuals from diverse backgrounds with unique challenges related to their adductor muscles. One such case involves a middle-aged athlete who suffered from chronic adductor strain due to overtraining. Through a targeted massage therapy regimen focusing on effleurage and petrissage strokes, combined with myofascial release techniques, the athlete experienced significant relief from pain and improved flexibility, allowing them to resume training with reduced risk of re-injury.

This case highlights the role of adductor massage in managing sports-related adductor issues and facilitating faster recovery.

Client testimonials provide firsthand accounts of the impact of adductor massage on their well-being. A client who struggled with persistent adductor tightness and discomfort, hindering their daily activities, shares their journey of seeking massage therapy. The incorporation of deep tissue massage for adductors, alongside stretching and strengthening exercises, resulted in a noticeable reduction in pain and increased range of motion. Such testimonials underscore the value of personalized massage interventions in addressing individual needs and enhancing quality of life.

Success stories in adductor massage reveal transformative outcomes achieved through consistent therapy and tailored treatment plans.

A case study involving a dancer grappling with adductor strains sheds light on the comprehensive approach adopted, incorporating myofascial release techniques and specialized stretches for adductor muscles. Over time, the dancer regained strength, flexibility, and confidence, ultimately returning to performances with improved performance and reduced risk of injury.

This narrative exemplifies the potential of adductor massage in optimizing musculoskeletal function and supporting career longevity in physically demanding fields.

These real-life examples and testimonials offer valuable insights and lessons for practitioners and individuals seeking to benefit from adductor massage therapies. Key learnings include the importance of personalized assessment and treatment plans, the integration of diverse massage techniques for holistic care, and the significance of patient education and compliance with home exercises.

By understanding these lessons and applying them in practice, professionals can optimize outcomes and empower clients to achieve lasting relief and functional improvement in adductor-related concerns.

Conclusion

In the journey of exploring adductor massage techniques, we've delved into the intricate anatomy of these muscles, understanding their pivotal role in movement, and recognizing the common issues and injuries they face. Moving beyond theory, we've discovered a treasure trove of benefits that adductor massage brings - from unlocking improved flexibility and range of motion to easing muscle tension and pain, all while elevating athletic performance and shielding against injuries.

Diving into the realm of massage therapy, we've navigated through the nuances of adductor massage, mastering the art of effleurage and petrissage strokes, exploring the depths of myofascial release techniques, and embracing the power of deep tissue massage for adductors. Alongside, we've prepared diligently, customizing each massage session to individual needs, ensuring a comfortable environment, and adhering to safety precautions with unwavering dedication.

But our journey doesn't end here. It extends into special considerations, where we leverage advanced massage tools, seamlessly integrate stretching and mobility exercises, and harmonize massage with other therapeutic modalities for holistic wellness. Post-massage care has become our mantra, advocating for hydration and nutrition, championing rest and recovery, and diligently monitoring progress to fine-tune our techniques for optimal results.

As we delve into advanced techniques and adaptations, we tailor adductor massage to sports-specific needs, unveil rehabilitation protocols for injuries, and unveil the blueprint for long-term maintenance and preventive strategies.

And amidst this rich tapestry of knowledge, we uncover the real gems - the case studies and success stories, where adductor massage transforms lives, earns heartfelt testimonials, and leaves an indelible mark on the landscape of wellness.

This isn't just about techniques; it's about a journey of transformation, empowerment, and resilience. It's about bridging the gap between theory and practice, between knowledge and application. So, as we conclude this exploration of adductor massage techniques, let's carry forward the torch of learning, innovation, and compassionate care, shaping a future where wellness thrives and bodies find their true strength.

www.ingramcontent.com/pod-product-compliance
Lightning Source LLC
Chambersburg PA
CBHW051719250726
48653CB00008B/3105